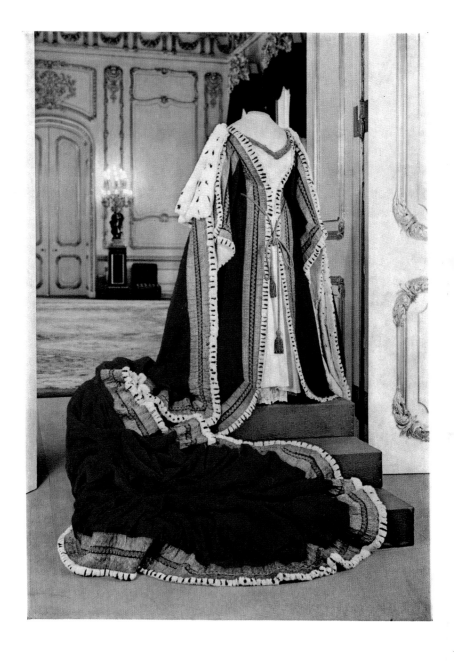

LONDON
MUSEUM

CORONATION COSTUME AND ACCESSORIES 1685-1953

LONDON
HER
MAJESTY'S
STATIONERY
OFFICE
1973

by Zillah Halls

with an introduction by Martin R. Holmes, FSA

SBN 11 290157 3

Coronation Costume and Accessories 1685-1953

Coronation Robes and Relics

By great good fortune, and by the generosity of royal and other donors, the London Museum collections now include examples of almost every type of ceremonial dress prescribed for English coronations over the last century and a half, and one or two individual pieces that are older still. The three sets of robes—crimson, cloth-of-gold and purple velvet—worn by the sovereign, the dresses and trains of queens consort, the uniforms worn by pages, privy councillors, court officials and great civic dignitaries, and even the empty frames of sovereigns' and consorts' crowns, are all represented, and combine to illustrate most expressively the development and significance of the ceremony.

One early feature of it, now long abandoned, is represented in the Museum by the embroidered velvet covering of the regalia-table that used to be set up in Westminster Hall (no 3). It was here that the peers of England assembled, from Norman times onward, to receive the new king before his consecration, and to show their acceptance of him by ceremonially raising him among them and seating him on the King's Bench. Only when this had been done was word sent to the Abbey—not yet a national institution, but the private church of a great medieval monastery. The abbot and monks of Westminster would then come to the Hall, attending the prelates who were to officiate and bringing with them the various articles of the Regalia, which were duly set out on a table before the king. From here they would be delivered to the great officers of State appointed to carry them, and the procession would make its way on foot from the Hall to the Abbey for the actual service of consecration, returning eventually for the splendours of the Coronation Banquet.

After the Reformation, the dean and chapter took over the functions of the abbot and his clergy. The ritual went on under their auspices, and the table-cover appears to have been used at the coronations of the first four kings of the house of Hanover. The Coronation of George IV, however, was so fantastically elaborate and expensive that his brother the Duke of Clarence, on succeeding him as William IV, was at one time reluctant to have a coronation ceremony at all. Eventually the religious service was retained, but the assembly in Westminster Hall beforehand, and the subsequent feasting, were abandoned and have not been revived.

The true focal point of the service is, and always has been, the moment of consecration and anointing by the officiating prelate, traditionally the Archbishop of Canterbury, Primate of All England. It is for this that the new king or queen puts off the crimson robes of entry, and it is only after this, and by virtue of this, that the royal ornaments may be assumed in succession till at last the wearer stands robed and crowned in front of the altar, ready to be 'lifted' into the throne and to receive the homage of the bishops and peers.

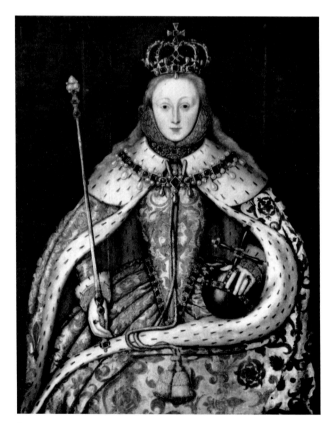

Queen Elizabeth I in her coronation robes, 1559. British School (Warwick Castle).

St Edward's Robes

The ensigns of royalty have consisted, from very early times, of ring, sword, crown, sceptre and 'rod of justice and equity', to which were added, in the twelfth century, the 'armills', or bracelets, and the imperial mantle. Further elaboration is however found a little later on, in two famous fourteenth-century manuscripts at Westminster, the Lytlington Missal, made for Abbot Nicholas de Lytlington about 1380, and the splendidly-illuminated Order of Service of about the same date, known as *Liber Regalis* – the Book Royal. Here, for the first time, we find a carefully-specified list of the vestments to be put on the new monarch immediately after the Anointing. First comes the *colobium sindonis*, a linen garment 'after the manner of a dalmatic', next, a long tunic wrought with figures in gold before and behind, and then the stockings or buskins, the sandals and the spurs of knighthood. The sword is girded on, and is followed by the delivery of the armills already mentioned, and the text contains an unusually elaborate explanation of their arrangement. They are to be suspended around the wearer's neck like a stole, hanging over both shoulders to the elbows, and are to be secured to his arms at the elbows by silken laces. In other words, the massive bracelets of gold are prevented from slipping down by being fastened to a band of fabric that goes over neck and shoulders like a very short stole, and is hidden, in a moment, by the imperial mantle, the next garment to be put on.

All this is a great elaboration on the earlier, simpler Orders of Service, but a memorandum in the Public Record Office, a little earlier in date, indicates the reason for it. This document is a schedule of procedure for a coronation, apparently that of Edward I, and contains references, for the first time, to the cult of the Confessor. In the Coronation Oath the new king now swears to guarantee the laws and customs granted 'by the glorious King St Edward'. After the Anointing, he is to put on 'the coat of St Edward which is at Westminster', later on he is invested with 'St Edward's Ring', and it is in his reign, too, that we first find reference to the continued existence of St Edward's Crown.

The explanation is quite a simple one, for the document means precisely what it says. Henry III, in his veneration for the Confessor, had not only demolished the main part of the Abbey Church and rebuilt it in a more up-to-date and splendid style, but he had taken St Edward's body from its tomb and transferred it, in 1269, to the great shrine behind the High Altar, where it still rests. In the process, the crown and vestments of the corpse had been retained in the abbey treasury as relics of the saint, finding a place, in due course, in the actual rite of coronation. The newly-anointed king, when receiving the conventional symbols of his office, was thenceforth invested in the actual garments and ornaments of the traditional 'good old king' who was regarded by this time as the ideal ruler and lawgiver of England. Being relics of the saint, the objects were abbey property which must naturally be given back as soon as possible after the service, so arrangements had to be made for the new king to change into something else for his return in procession to Westminster Hall. Even after the dissolution of the monastery of Westminster, and its reconstitution as a collegiate church, they continued to play their part in the service, being taken off at the end and delivered to the dean, as in former years they had been delivered to the abbot.

Charles I was the last king to be invested in St Edward's robes. After his execution, the treasury at Westminster was plundered, the saint's crown and staff were stripped of their jewels and broken up, and the robes, buskins, shoes, gloves,

Coronation of James II, 1685. Engraving by Sandford (London Museum).

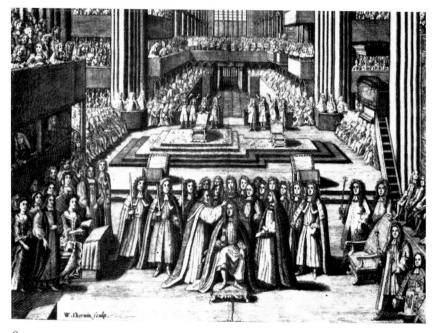

W. Sherwin sculp.

swords of state and St Edward's ivory comb were valued at £4 10s 6d in all, and pass into oblivion. New robes had to be made at the Restoration, appearing in rubrics as 'ye Robes, yt are called S. Edward's', but by this time their original position as permanent possessions of the Abbey had been misunderstood. Instead of calling on the abbey authorities, as heretofore, to produce the robes, each succeeding sovereign had a new set of golden vestments made for him, surrendered it in due course to the dean, and never saw it again. Many of the brocaded copes worn by canons of Westminster in living memory were once the mantles of Stuart and Hanoverian kings. One pair, indeed, can be identified, by their exact correspondence in material, design and construction, as those made for the unique joint coronation of William and Mary. In contrast to the seventeenth-century copes made for the abbey dignitaries, these are all of flowered brocade without embroidery, and in cut and construction they follow the lines laid down in Francis Sandford's contemporary account of the arrangements made for the coronation of James II in 1685, when the eagle-patterned mantle illustrated in his pages was not, in fact, ready in time, and was replaced by one originally triangular in form and made from strips of purple and gold brocade.

Coronation of George IV, 1821. Detail from aquatint by Dubourg (London Museum).

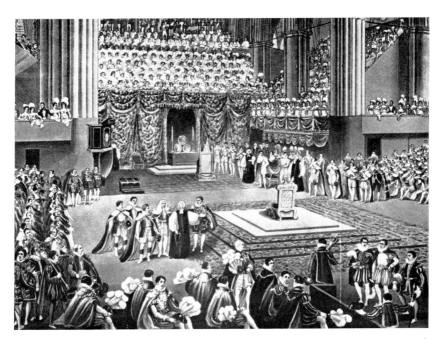

The splendid mantle of George IV was not made into a cope for the shoulders of any Westminster dignitary. The dean and prebendaries claimed their perquisites as usual, but though the cord and tassels of the king's mantle remain in the private possession of one of the dean's descendants, the mantle itself was sold, and it was only in the present century that it was rediscovered, purchased and presented to the Crown by a private donor. Since then it has been used at the Coronation of King George V and those of his successors, and it is now to be seen in the new Jewel House at the Tower.

Meanwhile, new sets of St Edward's Robes had to be made in succession for Queen Victoria and King Edward VII. Queen Victoria's imperial mantle (no 14, Plate 4) was made of the same fabric as that of George IV, with its roses, thistles and shamrocks in colour against a golden background patterned with eagles, crowns and fleurs-de-lys. Its sloping, rounded outlines and heavy bullion fringe give it a somewhat shawl-like appearance, but the rubric of the queen's coronation service alludes to it, quite inaccurately, as the 'dalmatic robe'. It is the sleeved supertunica worn under it, and still exhibited with it, that approximates a little more closely to the dalmatic form.

This time the royal robes remained in the royal possession, though the abbey authorities put up a brisk fight for some of their perquisites – as is demonstrated by a lively correspondence, now in the Public Record Office, between the Lord Chamberlain and the sub-dean, the redoubtable Lord John Thynne, both of whom laid claim to the silver inkstand used for the signing of the Coronation Oath. The robes made for the nineteen-year-old Queen Victoria, however, would hardly serve for the coronation of the older and ampler Edward VII more than sixty years afterwards. Mantle and supertunica (no 23) had to be made anew, with the decoration carried out in embroidery instead of brocade, and the only piece of the older vestments which could be adapted was the Coronation Stole. The symbols of England, Scotland and Ireland, the silver eagles and small open crowns between them, and the rectangular panels at either end with the Cross of St George, were detached from the short stole, still not much more than elbow-length, illustrated in Hayter's portrait of the Queen, and were laid down, much more widely spaced, on a longer strip of fabric that gave the stole a far closer resemblance to its ecclesiastical counterpart.

This gave support to the popular fallacy that the rite of coronation conferred some kind of ecclesiastical status, and the presence of the stole was called in evidence to prove the similarity of the rite to the consecration of a bishop. Its function as a band to support the armills had long been forgotten, the name armill was mistakenly applied to the strip of fabric itself, and though the doctrine of the king's being 'both layman and clerk' has been satisfactorily exploded by ecclesiological writers, the stoles of succeeding sovereigns have continued to be made in the proportions of the familiar church vestment.

Processional Robes

The king or queen regnant comes to the Abbey in parliament robes of crimson, which are taken off before the Anointing and carried away into St Edward's Chapel. Originally they became the perquisite of the monk who removed them; in later years this duty, and the right of retaining the king's body-garments, devolved upon the Lord Great Chamberlain. The coronation suit of George IV (no 5, Plate I) thus came into the family of the Earl of Ancaster, who generously deposited it on loan in the Museum. The traditional form of such robes is laid down by Sandford in his work already cited, and shows that there was some conscious archaism in their design, as they were obviously intended to reproduce the fashions of the Middle Ages, notably by the inclusion of a velvet surcoat with long hanging sleeves, slit to let out the hand and forearm, and a caped hood lying flat upon the shoulders.

George IV with trainbearers, 1821. Engraving by E. Scriven (London Museum).

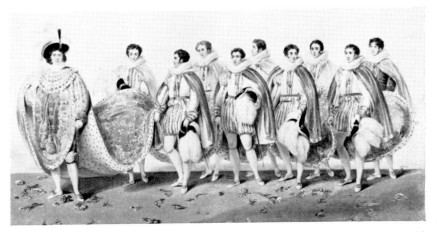

11

Not much more than a hundred years later, however, the fashion had changed, and by the third quarter of the eighteenth century the tendency in archaic or fancy dress was to imitate the modes of the early seventeenth. Gustavus III of Sweden had devised a national court costume of slashed doublet, short cloak and ruff; Charles Kemble compiled a stage wardrobe of mixed Elizabethan, Jacobean and Caroline fashions, and used it to depict English historical costume in general. Gainsborough, in 1770, painted young Jonathan Buttall in blue 'Van Dyck' costume, and at the coronation of George IV in 1821 the court and council were dressed in doublet and hose after a fashion ascribed indiscriminately to Holbein and Henri IV of France. The gentlemen-at-arms were resplendent in red and blue velvet, gold braid and a regular armoury of gilt buttons, the privy council had more-or-less Elizabethan costumes of blue and gold (no 7), the peers wore white and gold in the same style (still to be seen, under the mantles of the various Orders, in the first act of *Iolanthe*), and the king was similarly dressed, but in doublet and hose of cloth-of-silver under a wonderful garment of crimson and gold.

This suit (no 5, Plate I) pays eye-service, one may say, to the early regulations, as its velvet sleeves are detached and hang empty from the shoulders, but its cut is that of a fashionable court coat, fitting the body as creaseless as a glove. Comparison of the narrowness of the shoulders with the immense girth of the neck shows that the king must have been a slightly-built man before he ran to seed, and the amount of corseting and constriction that must have been necessary to get him into these garments fully accounts for the recorded fact that he used up nineteen pocket-handkerchiefs in the course of the Homage alone, the page who carried them reporting afterwards that he 'was more like an Elephant than a man'. The blaze of golden embroidery suggests that the wearer was determined at all costs to eclipse the sensation caused, some fifteen years before, by the splendour of Napoleon's Coronation as Emperor of the French, and the crimson parliament robe that went with it was quite as gorgeously ornamented. This, and its purple counterpart, were retained by the king, and were ultimately sold, after his death, to the indefatigable Mme Tussaud, in whose establishment they draped, for many years, the waxen figures of the last two Hanoverian kings of England.

Queen Victoria's crimson robes (frontispiece) resembled, in cut, those worn by Queen Adelaide as Queen Consort seven years before and, it would seem, by tragedy queens in general on the English stage. A tinsel picture of Mrs West playing Elvira in *Pizarro* about 1820 shows an exactly similar design,

A Privy Councillor at the Coronation of George IV, 1821. Engraving by E. Scriven (London Museum).

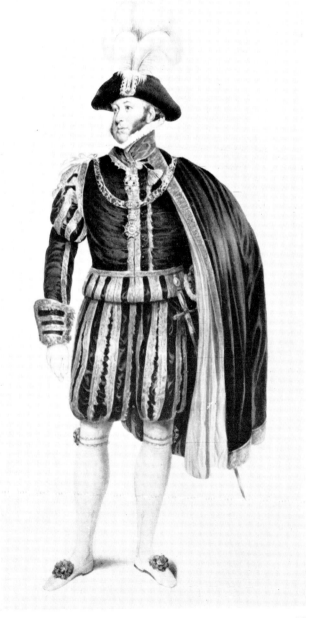

with its narrow waist, open front and hanging sleeves open to the shoulder, in a style popularly associated with the Middle Ages. A point that appears to have been unfortun arely overlooked, however, is the fact that whereas a queen consort retains her robes unchanged throughout the ceremony and an actress can change, when necessary in the comparative privacy of her dressing-room, a queen regnant has to be disrobed of her crimson velvet in the face of the whole congregation and, with this costume, that simply cannot be done. Like its theatrical prototype, the dress opens down the back of the bodice, its supposedly open front being stitched firmly into position, and having freed herself from the bodice and sleeves, the wearer has either to have the dress hauled over her head or to let it drop to the ground and step out of it in whatever she is wearing underneath. As it was, the queen had to retire from sight into St Edward's Chapel for the purpose, and duly reappeared already vested in some of St Edward's Robes, leaving only the mantle to be ceremonially put upon her by the dean.

The Robes of Entry of later sovereigns are represented only by one small but interesting item. Associated with the crimson robe worn by King George V as Prince of Wales at his father's coronation is a flat cap of crimson velvet trimmed with a stiff band of ermine, but the association is one of ideas only, based on correspondence of colour and material. That velvet cap (no 45) shows no sign of having been at any time the lining of a crown, certainly not the single-arched crown of a Prince of Wales. Its proportions and decorations suggest that it was the flat Cap of Estate that the King wore with his parliament robes when formally entering the Abbey for his own coronation, and laid aside for ever when he bared his head preparatory to receiving the holy oil.

There is nothing very striking about the state robes of Edward VII and George V (nos 24, 42). Each of them was cut like a full semicircular cloak, extending backwards into a train long enough to need nine pages to carry it. The George V robe is caught back, at about waist level, with bows of white satin ribbon, allowing a sight of the gold-braided purple surcoat worn beneath it; but the fuller figure of Edward VII would have called for no such emphasis, and his mantle accordingly falls unchecked from neck to hem.

Peeresses at the Coronation of William IV, 1831. Coloured engraving (London Museum).

Queens consort would appear, from the eighteenth century onwards, to have followed their own tastes in personal adornment, apart from the actual crown and the purple robe like a court train. Queen Adelaide wore, as we have seen, robes of the fashion associated with stage queens rather than that prescribed by the seventeenth-century heralds. Queen

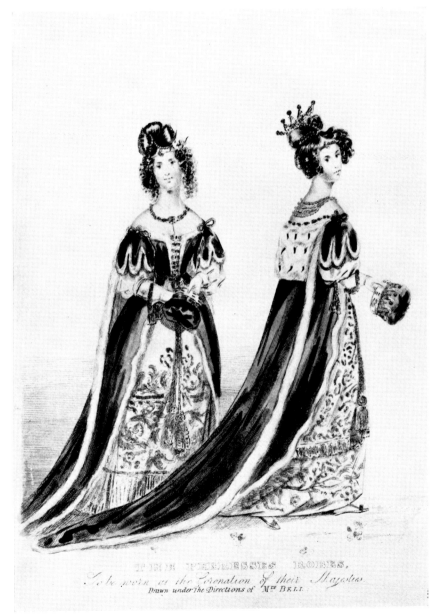

THE PEERESSES ROBES.
To be worn at the Coronation of their Majesties.
Drawn under the Directions of Mᵈ BELL.

Alexandra's high-standing wired collar (no 30, Plate 6) has a certain affinity with the Scandinavian and 'Henri IV' conventions already mentioned, not to speak of one of the last stage costumes worn by Adelina Patti in 1895 and also in the Museum's collection; but in other respects her gold gown with its overdress of embroidered net, is typical of the elaborate court dresses of the opening of the present century. Queen Mary's coronation dress (no 52, Plate 11) is of the characteristic 'princess' cut, its front stiff with gold and silver embroidery and a minute handkerchief-pocket incorporated in a vertical seam and ingeniously hidden by the embroidered pattern. Their purple robes (nos 29, 50, Plates 6, 11) hang from the shoulders like court trains, as does that of HM Queen Elizabeth the Queen Mother (no 67, Plate 20) and there has been no suggestion of a formal under-gown of archaic cut since the Coronation of Queen Adelaide as Consort in 1831.

For peeresses, however, the form long remained as prescribed by James II, through his Earl Marshal, in 1685. The close bodice, short sleeves ending in a scalloped border, and the scalloped or undulating edge to the skirt worn open over a contrasting petticoat (nos 80, 87, Plate 23) have shown little variation in two centuries-and-a-half. In 1952 a simplified version was authorised, with a shorter train, no sleeves and a round velvet cap instead of a coronet, for those below the rank of countess, and both types are now represented in the collections (nos 80, 87, 89, Plates 23, 24).

Crowns and Coronets

Of the Museum's six royal crown-frames, three were made for the coronations of consorts, one for the use of the king on his return to Westminster Hall, and two have performed the function of St Edward's Crown and been used for the actual coronation and investiture. All have been denuded of their jewels, but two have been reset with pastes, some of them being of exceptionally fine quality.

The oldest, and smallest, was originally made in 1685 for the crowning of Mary of Modena, Consort of James II (no 1). The holes in its rim correspond with the settings shown in Sandford's illustration of it, but are now concealed by the elaborate scrolled overlay of silver (later set with large eighteenth-century pastes) that must have been put on when the crown was used for the Coronation of Caroline of

Anspach, Consort of George II, in 1728. The arches have been cut through and re-riveted, indicating that this crown had been used, in the interim, as the single-arched crown of a Prince of Wales, and worn as such, at the Coronation of George I, by the prince who succeeded him as George II.

A large and elaborate crown, for many years incorrectly associated with Charles II, is now known to have been made for George I in 1715 as a Crown of State, and worn in that capacity by his son and great-grandson (no 2). George IV, however, had a new crown, in an open design of oak-leaves and acorns (no 4). This, too, was originally meant to be a Crown of State only, but when the time came it was used throughout, usurping the functions of St Edward's Crown. William IV was crowned with it likewise, but another new crown was made for the Coronation of his niece Queen Victoria in 1838 (no 12, Plate 3a). This also was used both as a coronation crown and a Crown of State, being lighter and easier to wear than the golden Crown of St Edward, still in the Tower. For this reason it was used again for the crown-ing of Edward VII, who was still weak from a serious illness, and it was King George V, in 1911, who revived the use of St Edward's Crown.

Coronation of George V, 1911. Detail from oil by J. H. F. Bacon (Royal Collection, on loan to the House of Lords).

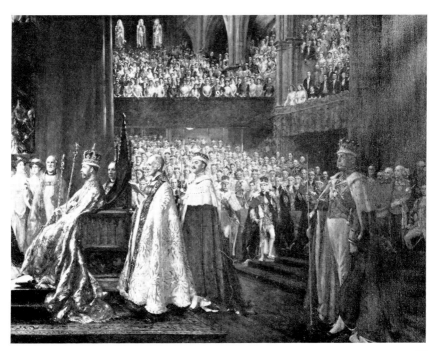

By 1937, when preparations were being made for the Coronation of King George VI, it was felt that Queen Victoria's crown, by this time nearly a hundred years old, was getting too frail to be safely used. The present State Crown was accordingly made, and the empty frame of its predecessor remained in the hands of the crown jewellers till its fragments were presented to the Museum and reassembled in its workshops by the technical staff.

A point worth remembering is that the diamonds and pearls worn in a consort's coronation crown were customarily hired, not bought, since they were needed for a few hours only, a lesser crown, or Crown of State, being worn on other ceremonial occasions. After the ceremony the stones went back to the jewellers and were replaced, if the crown was to be displayed, by pastes, crystals or semi-precious stones. Queen Adelaide had disliked this idea, and the crown that had been made for her was set with jewels that were her own personal property. Queen Alexandra was the last consort to be crowned in hired diamonds, and the tall, graceful crown that was designed for her (no 26, Plate 7a) was re-set with pastes before she graciously presented it, and the dress and accessories worn with it, to the newly-formed London Museum. (On other state occasions it appears that she wore a small diamond crown made for Queen Victoria and still to be seen in the Tower).

A noticeable feature of the coronets made for women is their small size. The coronet of a peeress is, in its design and ornamentation, similar to that of a peer of equal rank, but is only some five inches across. So, it will have been noticed, are the Mary of Modena crown and the crown-frame made for Queen Adelaide. These two early examples would perch in quite a becoming manner on the high-piled hairdressing of their day, but by the time of Queen Victoria's accession the fashion had changed. Hair was dressed close to the head, with a knot at the back, and a crown, wreath or tiara would therefore be expected to correspond more closely with the proportions of the head itself. Preliminary enquiry at the Tower had produced the report that the queen's crowns in its Jewel House were 'small and in poor condition', and the crown made for the young queen was consequently as large as a man's, a fact which enabled it later to be worn, in succession, by her son and grandson.

The coronets of peeresses, however, remained small, and for a doctrinal reason. It is only in comparatively recent years that the Church of England has ceased to insist on compliance with St Paul's injunction to women to keep their heads covered when engaged in prayer. A peeress, at a coronation, does not put on her coronet until the queen herself is crowned, but it was inconceivable that she should be allowed to remain bareheaded through the earlier part of the service. The queen consort herself, when there was one, went to her coronation in the 'diadem' of gold, velvet and diamonds first made for Mary of Modena, worn by her and her successors and still preserved in the Jewel House. For her, with her attendant ladies to help her, it was possible to take off the earlier headdress before the imposition of the crown, but the peeresses, having no attendants, could do nothing of the sort. The regulations laid down, accordingly, that veils and tiaras should be worn, to constitute an orthodox head-covering, and the coronet should be small enough to be put on, when the time came, *inside* the circle of the tiara without disturbing it or the wearer's coiffure (no 87). An ingenious device to be found on some peeresses' coronets was the provision of small sliding rods, like miniature hatpins, which were permanently attached to the rim of the coronet. These, when it was put on, could be thrust home through the piled-up hair beneath, and would serve to ensure, to a great degree at least, the steadiness of the coronet and the wearer's peace of mind.

Associated Pieces

Certain objects connected with the coronation ceremony have traditionally become the perquisites of the Abbey or the royal household. It is from a former Lord Chamberlain that the Museum acquired the cushion on which Queen Victoria had knelt for her anointing (no 16). The cloth-of-gold canopy held over her at that moment had been an abbey perquisite, but must have been among the material 'redeemed' by a money payment, since it appeared unexpectedly in a London sale-room not so very long ago (no 15). The Dymoke Armour in the Museum recalls the ceremony of the Challenge, in which a member of the Dymoke family maintained his tenure of the Manor of Scrivelsby in Lincolnshire by riding into Westminster Hall in armour from the royal armoury, after the first course of the Coronation Banquet, and offering to meet in combat anyone bold enough to deny the new king's right to the crown and throne of England. He customarily claimed, and sometimes obtained, the armour as part of his fee, and the suit in the Museum is apparently the one worn, and in due course claimed, by Sir John Dymoke in respect of his service at the coronation of George III.

Another manorial tenure was confirmed by service of a different kind. When the king was anointed on the hands as well as the head, he was accustomed to put on linen gloves and a linen coif immediately afterwards, to cover the oil. Later in the ceremony his right-hand glove had to be removed when he was invested with the coronation ring, and the Lord of the Manor of Farnham Royal 'did service' for his manor by providing a new glove for the king's right hand and, if required, supporting his arm to bear the weight of the sceptre. In 1541 the Earl of Shrewsbury exchanged the manor of Farnham Royal for that of Worksop, and the service was done thereafter in respect of the latter manor until it in its turn became extinct in the last reign (nos 25, 47, 66). At the last coronation, therefore, an individual had to be nominated by the Crown to perform the service irrespective of any manorial tenure, and the office was performed, accordingly, by Lord Woolton.

Other individual items in the collection illustrate this or that point of ritual or tradition. A small bag of crimson velvet once held the 'mark of gold' brought by Queen Victoria as her coronation offering (no 21); the stiff embroidered purse carried by the attendant upon the Lord Chancellor marks that dignitary's function as Keeper of the Great Seal; the splendid robe of a Lord Mayor (no 60), of crimson velvet barred with ermine and gold lace, is in its turn a token of his duty to attend the service carrying the City Sceptre of crystal and gold, reputedly the oldest staff of office still in use. The very sword-hilts of the court pages show by their horse-head pommels that they are under the authority of the Master of the Horse, who has just such a pommel on the hilt of his own sword (no 59). Among all this elaboration, however, the ceremony still primarily consists of its three main sections—acclamation, consecration and investiture—and in this respect is still essentially the rite with which William of Normandy was crowned King of England in the Confessor's new church at Westminster just over nine hundred years ago.

MARTIN R. HOLMES.

Plates

Plate 1
Coronation dress
of George IV,
1821 (no 5)

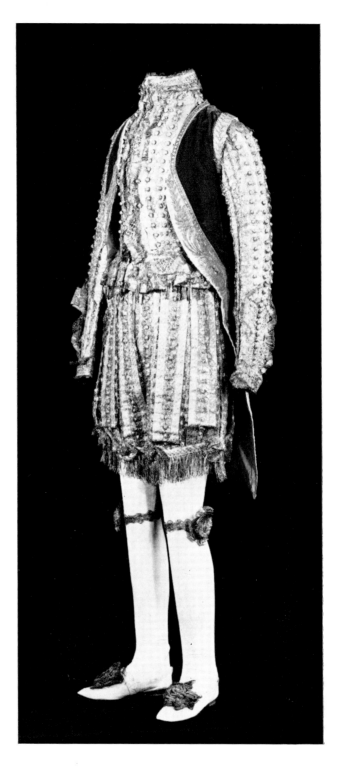

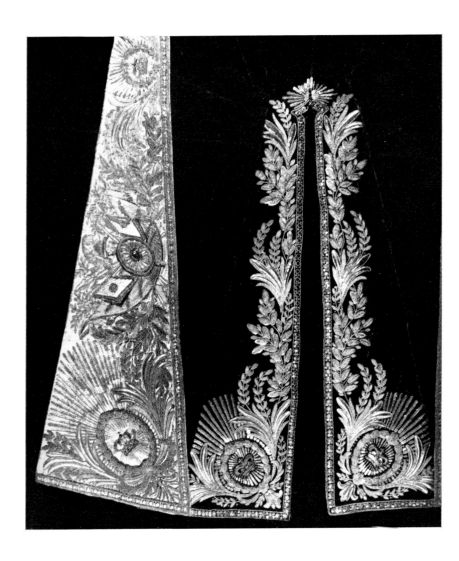

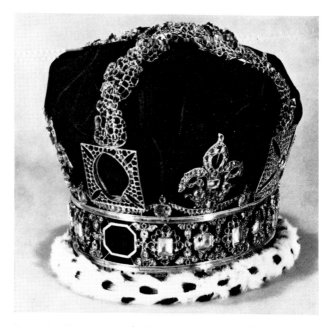

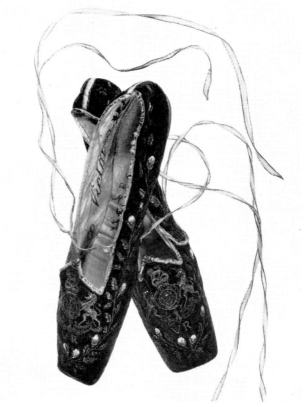

24

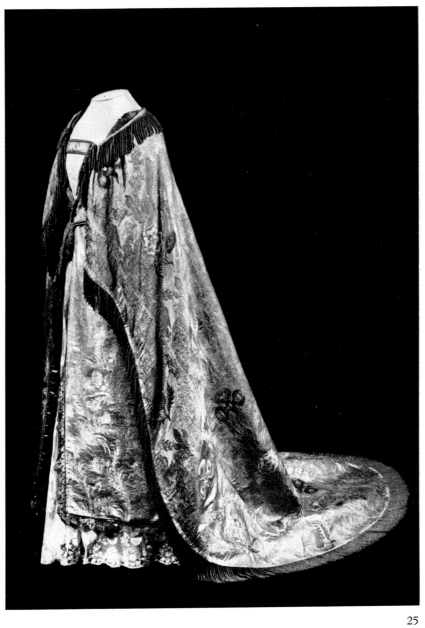

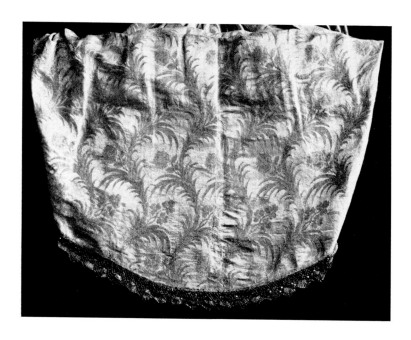

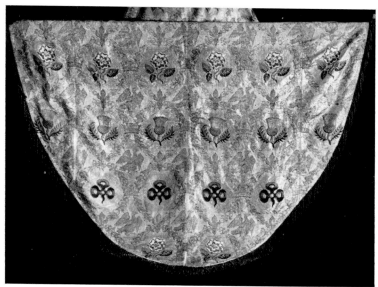

Plate 6   Photograph of Queen Alexandra in her coronation robes, 1902 (no 29)

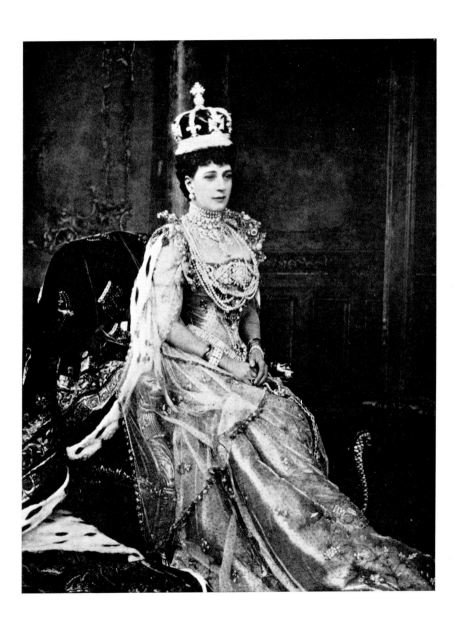

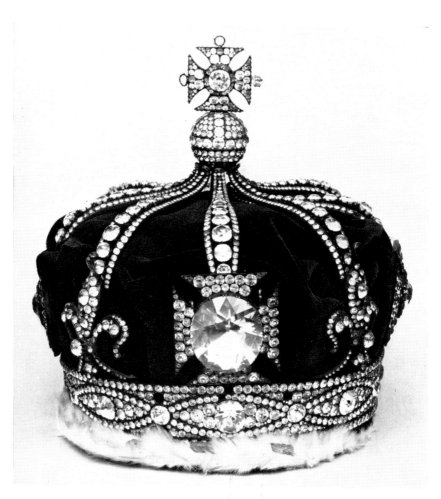

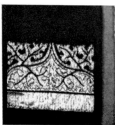 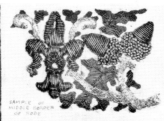 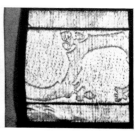

Plate 8a   Queen Alexandra's coronation gloves, 1902 (no 31)

Plate 8b   Detail of the embroidery on Queen Alexandra's coronation
                 dress, 1902 (no 30)

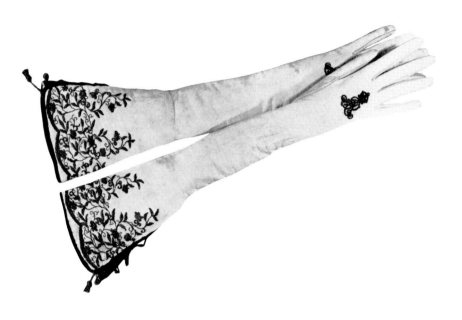

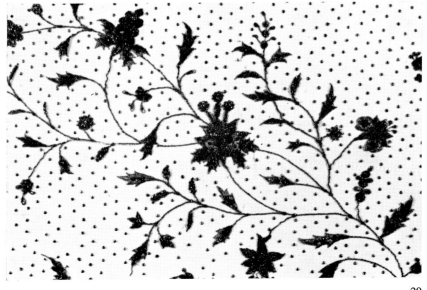

Plate 9a   Detail from the dress worn by Queen Mary as Princess of Wales at the Coronation of Edward VII, 1902 (no 35)

Plate 0b   Detail ot embroidery from the train belonging to the dress worn by Queen Mary as Princess of Wales at the Coronation of Edward VII, 1902 (no 35)

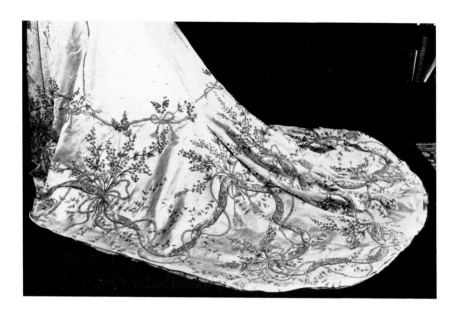

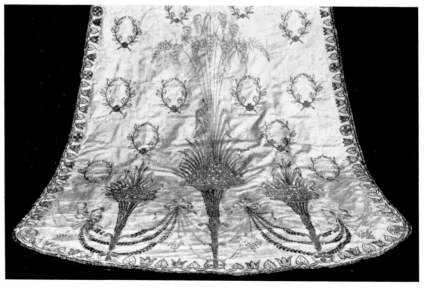

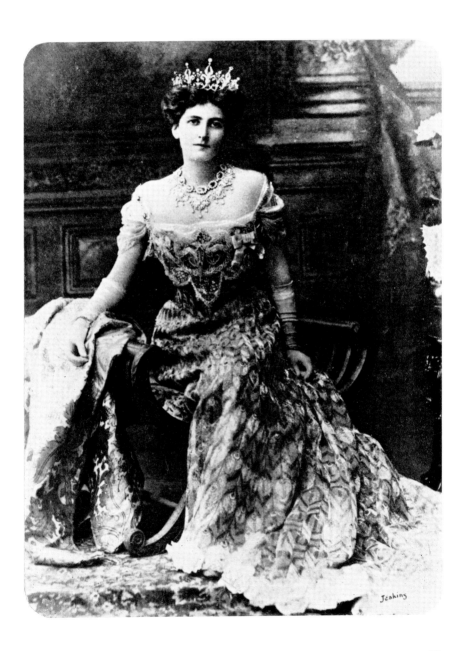

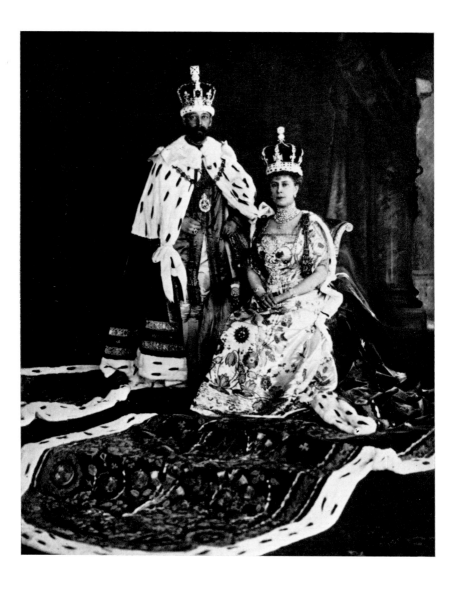

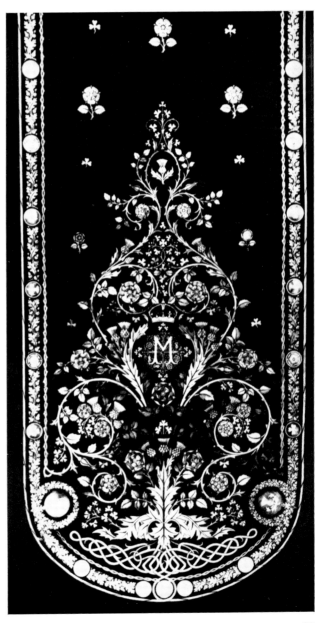

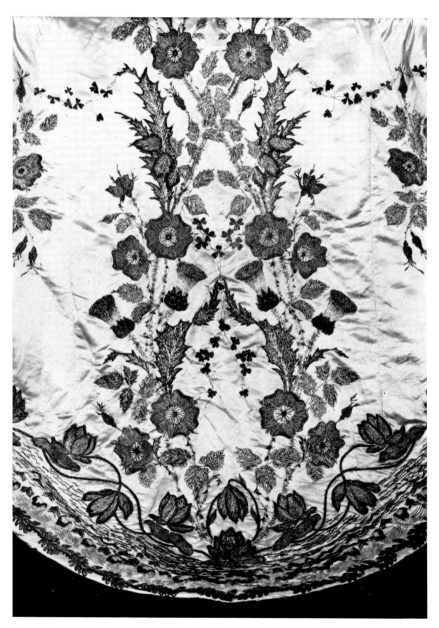

Plate 14
Samples of
embroidery for
Queen Mary's
coronation robe,
1911 (no 49)

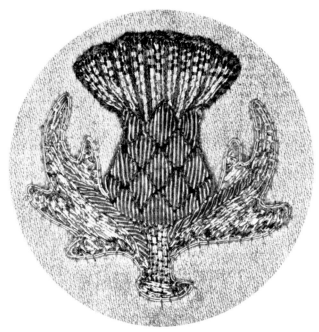

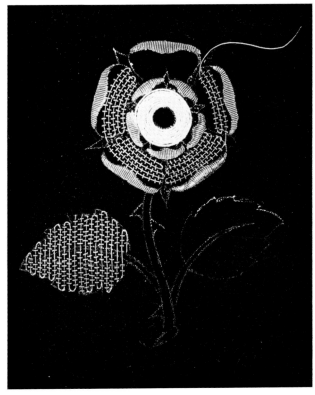

35

Plate 15   Gold girdle and stole of George V, 1911 (no 46)

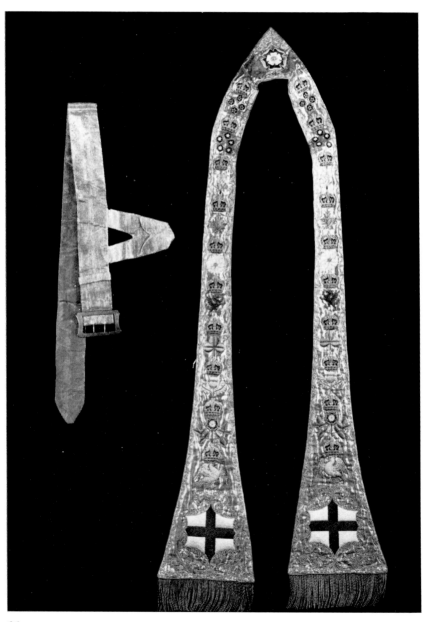

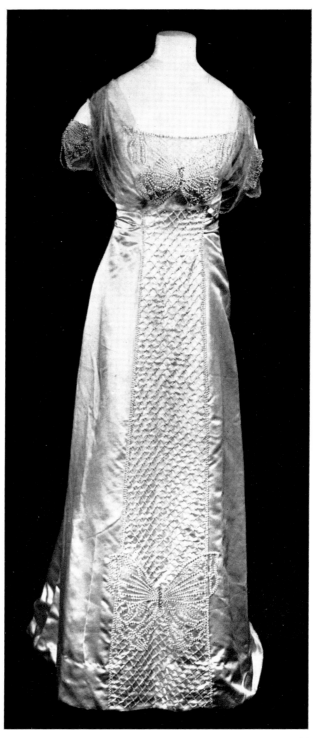

Plate 16
Dress worn by one of the train-bearers of Queen Mary, 1911 (no 55).

Plate 17   Dress worn at the Delhi Durbar, 1912 (no 64)

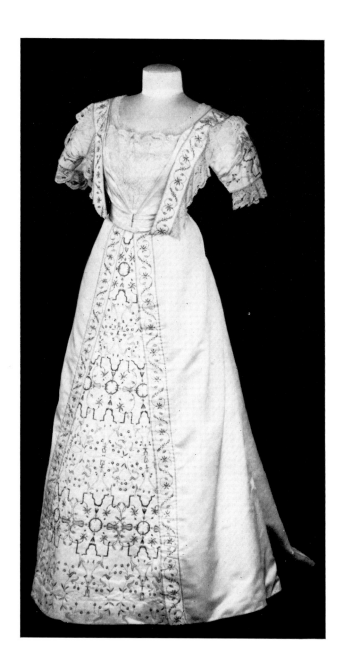

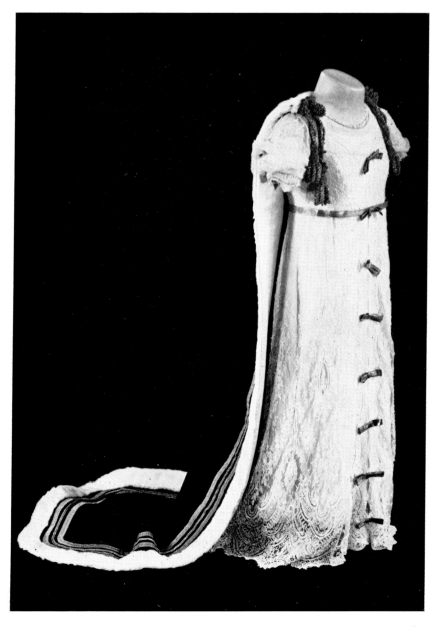

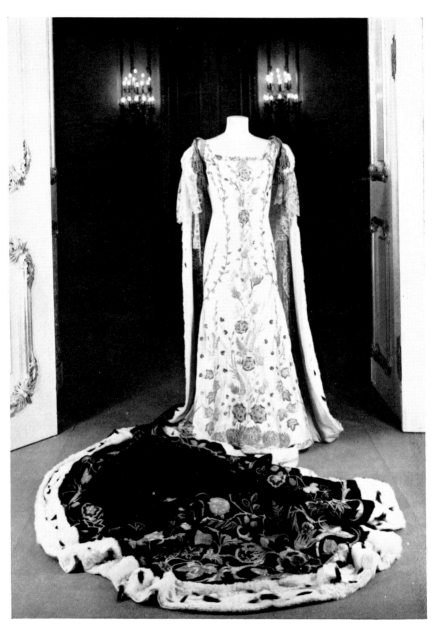

Plate 20 Coronation robe of Queen Elizabeth the Queen Mother, 1937 (no 67)

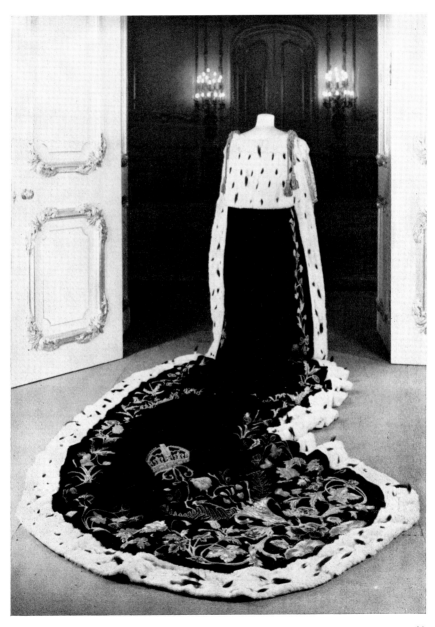

Plate 21   Dress worn by the Duchess of Kent, 1937 (no 77)

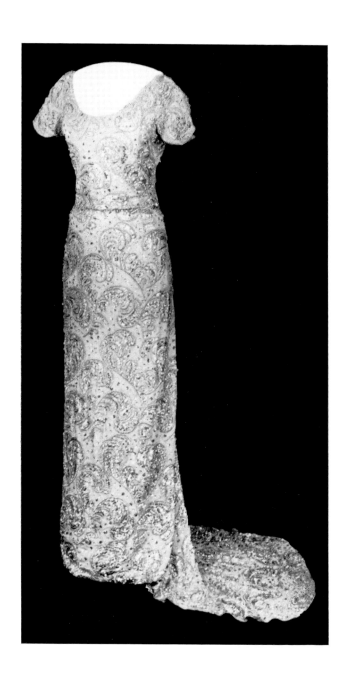

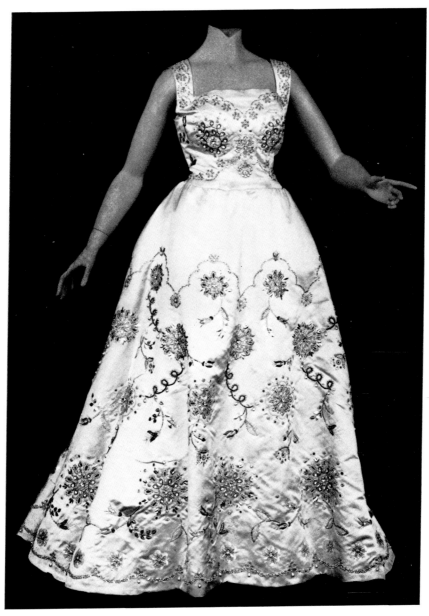

Plate 23   Robes of a peeress, old-style (no 87)

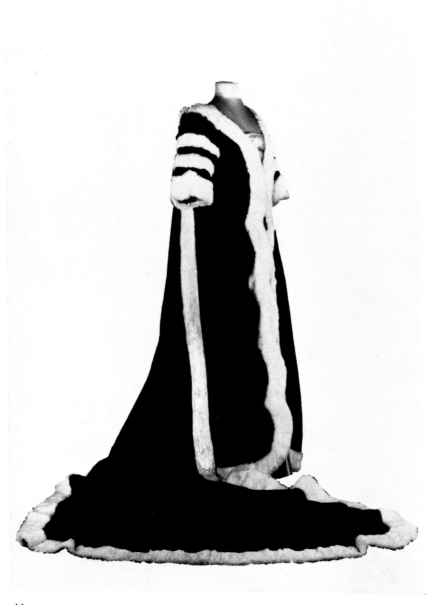

Plate 24 Robes of a peeress, new-style, 1953 (no 89).

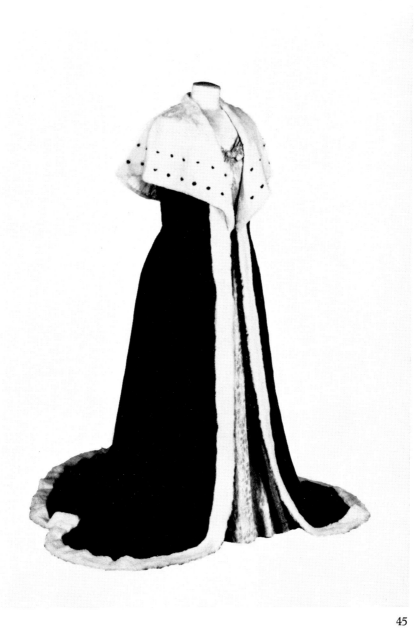

Plate 25
Dress worn by
Lady Hutton,
1953 (no 86)

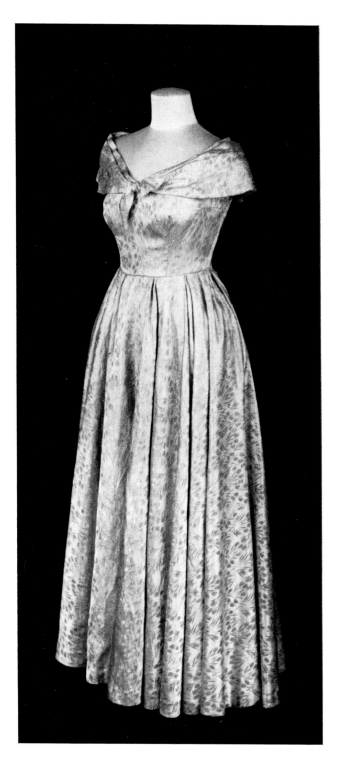

Catalogue

The Coronation of James II, 1685

1 The crown worn by Mary of Modena at the Coronation of
James II, 1685; it is a small crown of gold and silver, which
was reset for Queen Caroline of Anspach to wear at the
Coronation of George II in 1728; it had been worn at the
previous coronation, that of George I in 1715, by the Prince of
Wales. In its present form it is set with paste diamonds, with a
circlet of pearls round the edge; there is a crimson crown-cap,
and a white silk lining.
56.11

The Coronation of George I, 1715

2 The coronation crown of George I (subsequently worn by
George II and George III); consisting of a solid gold circlet
with crosses and fleurons, the circlet and arches set with
detachable silver and gilt jewel settings. The finial is missing
and the crown cap is a later replacement.
37.7/1

3 Table coverlet, made for the Coronation of George I, and
probably used by the three succeeding monarchs (George II,
George III, George IV); it was last used at George IV's
Coronation. The coverlet is rectangular, and made of crimson
velvet with a broad applied border of gold braid and in the
centre applied motifsGR, the crown, and the rose and thistle.
Condition: good but soiled and tarnished; cleaned in the
Museum
D 203

The Coronation of George IV, 1821

4 The coronation crown of George IV (subsequently used by
William IV); formed of a double circlet of gold, enclosing
openwork silver settings for jewels in a flower pattern; the
crosses and fleurons, the four arches (with an oak-leaf pattern),
and the finial, are of openwork silver to take jewels, This is the
largest of the royal crowns in the Museum; it has a dark blue
velvet crown-cap.
37.7/2

5   Coronation dress of George IV; this consists of a cloth-of-silver doublet and trunk hose, very lavishly trimmed with gold lace and gold braid; a sleeveless surcoat (with detached sleeves) of crimson velvet faced with silver and embroidered with gold; a sword belt of crimson velvet embroidered with gold; a pair of silver ribbon garters with trimming and rosettes of gold lace, and a pair of white kid shoes with red heels and gold lace rosettes.
Of all the surviving examples of coronation dress this is probably the most striking example of the combination, in one ceremonial dress, of personal idiosyncrasy, current fashion and ancient tradition. No British sovereign before or since has been crowned in an ensemble so closely akin to fancy dress though the possibility of European inspiration (e.g. the Coronation of Napoleon) cannot be discounted. The King was undoubtedly guided by his own personal taste but he was also well in line with current fashion which, in the years around 1820, favoured a harking-back to historically-inspired details, particularly those of Tudor and Stuart origin. In the lavish use of gold and silver George IV was again following his own taste, but the crimson surcoat was the traditional garment to be worn under the crimson parliament robe, worn by the sovereign for the approach to Westminster Abbey; the robe itself is preserved at Madame Tussaud's Ltd.
Condition: excellent; as in other examples surviving from this period, the metal lace and embroidery are quite free from tarnish
53.169/1-11   *Plates* 1, 2

6   Sword-belt worn by the Duke of Clarence (afterwards William IV) at the Coronation of George IV; crimson velvet with gold buckles and fittings.
Condition: good
59.28/3

7   Privy Councillor's dress worn by the Rt Hon George Canning at the Coronation of George IV. This consists of a doublet and trunk-hose, and a cloak, in a style very much in keeping with the King's own fancy-dress Tudor style of coronation dress. All three garments are made of blue satin, liberally trimmed with gold braid; the cloak is lined with crimson silk.
Condition: excellent
39.67/1-3

8   Uniform of the Harbinger of the Gentlemen Pensioners, worn at the Coronation of George IV by Col Samuel Wilson, who was also Harbinger at the Coronations of William IV and Queen Victoria. George IV, according to the donor of the uniform, ordered this suit to be made as an exact reproduction of the Harbinger's uniform worn at the Coronation of Henry VIII. This would not appear to be strictly true; nevertheless the garments are made in the same 'Tudor' style as the garments worn at the Coronation of George IV by the King

himself and by the Rt Hon George Canning. They consist of
trunk hose and doublet, a short cape, gloves and shoes. The
doublet and hose are of crimson velvet with puffed insertions
of grey-blue velvet, and liberal trimmings of gold braid with
gilt studs; the crimson velvet cape has similar trimming, and
long gold cord ties with gold tassels, and the white satin shoes
have large gold-trimmed rosettes.
Condition: good except for shoes, very worn and fragile
32.214

9   Tabard of a poursuivant, damask lined with red silk, bearing
the royal arms of the later Hanoverian sovereigns; the use of
damask (as opposed to satin) indicates the tabard of a
poursuivant; the presence of a crown over the Hanoverian
inescutcheon indicates a date after 1814, when the crown was
substituted for the Electoral hat. It appears likely that the
tabard was worn at the Coronation of George IV by Francis
Martin, FSA (1767-1841), who was appointed Windsor Herald
4 April 1819; also that he wore the tabard for the subsequent
Coronations of William IV and Queen Victoria before his
appointment as Norroy King of Arms, 5 February 1839.
Condition: fair; the woollen backing for the heraldic motifs
has suffered from moth damage
A 13815

The Coronation of William IV, 1831

10   Queen Adelaide's crown frame; this like George IV's crown
which was used again for the Coronation of William IV and
Queen Adelaide, is formed of a double circlet of gold,
enclosing silver settings for jewels. Again, the crosses,
fleurons, arches and finials are of openwork silver, to take
jewels; there is a crimson velvet crown-cap.
37.7/3

11   Bag, made of material from the coronation canopy of William
IV. The character of the material, woven entirely of gold
thread and strip and yellow silk, and the long gold fringe at
the base, are comparable with the coronation canopy of Queen
Victoria (no 15). The more flamboyant pattern of large rose
sprays is, despite William IV's distaste for ostentation, in
keeping with the aesthetic climate of the early 1830s, which
was more exuberant than that of the late 1830s when there
were already signs of the restraint, amounting almost to
severity, which was to characterise the early Victorian period.
Condition: of fabric, good
64.5

The Coronation of Queen Victoria, 1838

12   The Imperial State Crown of Queen Victoria; like the crowns
      of George IV and Queen Adelaide, this is formed of a double
      circlet of gold; the jewel-settings are again silver, and on the
      arches, supported by gold framework, they are in the form of
      oak-leaves. The finial is missing; the crimson velvet crown-
      cap and miniver circlet survived separately and were re-
      assembled in the Museum.
      58.74   36.112/1, 2   *Plate 3a*

13   The Parliament robe and surcoat of Queen Victoria. Both
      garments are of crimson velvet, with gold borders and an
      edging of ermine; the robe is also lined with ermine.
      The form of the surcoat is clearly related to contemporary
      fashion; it has a closely-fitting boned bodice fastening down
      the centre back; the centre front bodice section is of white
      satin, ending in a long pointed waistline. The skirt, full and
      gathered to the bodice, is open down the centre front; the
      wide hanging velvet sleeves are completely open from the
      shoulder, so that the small close-fitting undersleeves, very
      similar in shape to those of contemporary evening wear, are
      just visible. They are made of white satin covered with two
      layers of bobbin lace, one white, and covered by the other
      which is white and gold. The robe, with its shoulder-cape of
      white ermine, is hooked to the surcoat on the shoulders.
      Condition: good; this is the only coronation robe in the
      Museum which still retains its original, if somewhat torn,
      ermine, except for the shoulder-cape which has been replaced
      by later imitation ermine.
      48.14/12   *Frontispiece*

14   The gold supertunica and pallium of Queen Victoria. Both
      garments are of gold tissue woven with the national emblems.
      The supertunica, woven with the rose and thistle, is loose and
      open in front, with the full skirt gathered into the waist at the
      back; it has loose open sleeves very similar in cut to those of
      the crimson velvet surcoat; it is edged with gold lace, and
      lined with crimson satin. The pallium, its shape reminiscent
      of a cope and woven with the rose, thistle and shamrock, and
      the crown and eagle, has a similar satin lining, and gold fringe
      edging.
      Condition: good
      48.14/10, 11   *Plates 4, 5a, 5b*

15   The gold canopy and staves used for Queen Victoria's
      Coronation. The canopy consists of a rectangle of gold tissue,
      woven with silver floral sprays on a striped gold background;
      it is lined with silver tissue and edged with a gold fringe. The
      silver-mounted staves which supported the canopy are
      preserved with it in the Museum.
      Condition: good
      54.49

16 Altar cushion on which Queen Victoria knelt at her Coronation. The cushion is rectangular, and made of crimson satin with yellow cord edging; it is embroidered in one corner 'The Altar Cushion on which Queen Victoria knelt at her Coronation in Westminster Abbey July 28 1838'.
Condition: one side good, the other very worn
29.36/1

17 Shoes worn by Queen Victoria at her Coronation – purple velvet slippers embroidered with the royal arms in gold, and with rosebuds in gold thread and pink silk; lined with white satin embroidered with the rose, thistle and shamrock in coloured silks, and 'All Hail Victoria'.
Condition: good; gold thread rather tarnished
33.77/1   *Plate 3b*

18 Stocking worn by Queen Victoria at her Coronation; very fine cream silk, machine-knitted; the openwork fronts embroidered in coiled gold thread; the tops worked 'VICTORIA I REINE D'ANGLETERRE'.
Condition: fragile
33.77/2

19 Morse from Queen Victoria's coronation pallium. Gilt metal, later incorporated into a belt, but restored in the Museum to its original condition.
Condition: good, apart from alteration
52.141

20 Crown of a King-of-Arms, silver-gilt, in the form of acanthus-leaves above the motto 'MISERE. MEI : DEUS . SECUNDUM . MAGNAM . MISERICORDIAM. TUAM'; crimson satin crown-cap, ermine rim, gold finial, cream silk lining; the crown is in its own case. It was apparently worn at the Coronation of Queen Victoria, as it bears the hallmark 1838. It appears to have been made for Joseph Hawker, who was promoted to King-of-Arms from being a herald in that year. It subsequently belonged to S. E. Cokayne, Norroy King-of-Arms 1882, Clarenceaux 1894–1911; it was presumably therefore worn at the Coronations of Edward VII and George V.
Condition: good, apart from ermine, damaged by moth
56.191

21 Bag used at the coronation of Queen Victoria. Small square bag of red velvet, embroidered with oak sprays, in coiled gold thread; gold tassels, fringe edging and gold handle; lined with white silk.
Condition: good; metal slightly tarnished
D 278

The Coronation of Edward VII, 1902

22   Original tracing for the embroidery on Edward VII's supertunica, and design for his pallium (this design was not executed).
54.140/1, 2

23   The cloth-of-gold vestments (supertunica, pallium and stole) worn by Edward VII at his Coronation. The supertunica, of plain gold tissue, is in the form of a long-sleeved coat, without fastenings and almost without shaping; the only decoration is a border on the front edges, worked with laid orange-brown silk. The original design (no 22) shows an additional wider border, but there was no time to execute this. The supertunica is unlined, but the yellow silk on the reverse side of the fabric gives the impression of a lining. The pallium, like that of Queen Victoria, is lined with crimson satin, and it is richly patterned – the design is of roses, thistles, shamrocks, crowns, eagles, olive branches and passion flowers. The differences between this pallium and that of Queen Victoria are firstly the shape; Edward VII's is more cope-like than Queen Victoria's; also, whereas the pattern of the 1838 pallium is woven, the 1902 one is embroidered, by the Royal School of Needlework. The stole, too, is of gold tissue, lined with crimson satin, and embroidered. The design, worked mostly in laid silver thread, is of roses, crowns, thistles, shamrocks and eagles; each end is worked with a red cross on a silver ground.
Condition: the supertunica is well-preserved, but the pallium and the stole are badly tarnished and the embroidery faded
48.14/13, 14, 15

24   Royal robe worn by Edward VII on his return from the Abbey. This purple velvet robe is very similar, except in colour, to the Parliament robe of Queen Victoria (no 13). The gold braid border is almost identical; it too is edged with ermine and has an ermine shoulder-cape. It is not however lined with ermine; also, unlike Queen Victoria's robe, it is shaped to form a cape, almost meeting in front and falling to the ground, the back extended to form a long train.
Condition: fair; the gold braid is tarnished, and the ermine has been replaced by later imitation ermine
48.14/1 (formerly 33.213)

25   Coronation glove presented to Edward VII by the Lord of the Manor of Worksop. The glove is of white leather, with a coronet and the arms of Verdun embroidered on the back of the hand; the large stiffened gauntlet is lavishly embroidered with coiled gold thread and spangles with the Tudor rose, the shamrock, the thistle, and oak leaves and acorns, and is lined with crimson satin. The glove survives in its original case of crimson velvet lined with crimson quilted satin.
Condition: good; gold embroidery rather tarnished and soiled
48.14/2 (formerly 33.215)

26   The coronation crown of Queen Alexandra; a double circlet of gold wire, holding platinum settings for jewels, re-set with imitation stones; the crosses, fleurons, eight arches, and finial are all openwork silver, to take jewels; the finial with cross, is attached with a gold wire setting which enables it to be removed; there is a purple velvet crown-cap, and the original purple velvet case.
48.14/6 (formerly 33.214/4)   *Plate 7a*

27   Tracings for the embroidery on Queen Alexandra's coronation robe
54.140/3–17, 21, 22

28   Samples of the three borders of Queen Alexandra's coronation robe. The outer border (to which 222 embroidered gold roses were to be applied) and the inner border, are woven of gold thread and 'petunia' (i.e. purple with a hint of crimson) silk. The middle border, of oak sprays, fleurs-de-lis and crosses, is embroidered in various types of gold thread, and gold beads.
Condition: new
54.140/18–20   *Plate 7b*

29   Purple velvet robe worn by Queen Alexandra for her Coronation in 1902. The colour of the velvet is not the violet shot with crimson in the warp, traditional for a queen of England, but a different purple shade, chosen by the Queen and called 'petunia' by Princess Louise. There is an ermine shoulder-cape and lining, and three borders–the samples (no 28) show these in new condition. The embroidery on the end of the robe is symbolic of the British Empire, which appears in the form of a rose-tree, with shamrocks and thistles, springing from the Saxon crown, and with many fleurs-de-lis at the roots, to represent its Saxon and French origins. It culminates in the Star of India and the Royal Crown of 1902. The rest of the robe is sprinkled with crowns. As Queen Consort, not Queen of England in her own right, the Queen was not strictly speaking supposed to have all the royal emblems on her robe–for instance the Crown and the Star; she desired them however and the design incorporating them all was drawn by Mr Frederick Vigers, FRIBA, and executed by the Ladies' Work Society, presided over by Princess Louise; Miss Jessie Robinson's manuscript notes (54.140/83) have provided the information about the coronation robes of Queen Alexandra and Queen Mary. The gold borders were woven by Messrs Warner of Braintree; the velvet was woven by an old Huguenot weaver, M Dorée, and supplied by Messrs Marshall and Snelgrove, and the making-up of the robe was by Messrs Ede and Ravenscroft.
Condition: very poor. The velvet is split and the pile worn, and the embroidery very soiled and tarnished. The background of the embroidered borders has lasted better than the rest because it is a different more durable velvet
33.214/2   *Plate 6*

30 Dress worn by Queen Alexandra for her coronation in 1902; the dress is of gold tissue, under white net embroidered with gold spangles and gold and silver floral sprays. The long open hanging sleeves are of similar net; all the edges are trimmed with gold bobbin lace, and the wired outstanding collar is of gold bobbin lace with imitation pearl, diamanté and gilt decoration. The maker's label inside the waist reads 'Thorin-Blossier, 15 Rue Daunou, Paris'. The dress, though suitably magnificent for a coronation, shows little divergence from current fashion. Lady Curzon, wife of the Viceroy of India, supervised the weaving of the material and the working of the embroidery; the pattern of Indian flora has a very eastern character. It is not easy to see for certain whether the rose and thistle have in fact been incorporated in the design or not, despite the assurance of the account of the dress in the *Daily Telegraph* at the time of the Coronation that they were included. Subsequently Queen Mary, Queen Elizabeth the Queen Mother, and HM Queen Elizabeth II all wore, for their coronations, dresses embroidered with national emblems; these, also well represented in Queen Alexandra's robe (no 29) seem to have been absent from Queen Victoria's dress as far as can be seen from contemporary illustrations.

Queen Alexandra was 57 at the time of her Coronation; photographs taken of her at the time show her still to have been dazzlingly beautiful, and the waist measurement of the dress is 23 inches.

Condition: fair; the metal thread is rather tarnished, and the skirt has been relined

33.214/1 *Plates 6, 8b*

31 Gloves worn by Queen Alexandra at her Coronation in 1902; long white kid gloves with the wrist opening fastening with buttons and buttonholes; the crown and royal cypher are embroidered on the back of the hand, and the ends embroidered with a leaf pattern in coiled gold thread, and lined with purple velvet like that of the train. There is gold lacing at the outer arm. The gloves were made by the King's glovers, Messrs Harborow of New Bond Street.

Condition: good but rather soiled

33.214/3 *Plate 8a*

32 Shoes worn by Queen Alexandra at her Coronation in 1902; the shoes are of gold tissue, and the low fronts have a gold bow, and a crown and two interlaced 'A's embroidered mostly in gold and silver thread; the heels are of medium height.

Condition: poor

33.214/5

33 Crimson velvet robe worn by George V as Prince of Wales at the Coronation of Edward VII, 1902; a semicircular cape, gathered at the neck under the ermine shoulder-cape, speckled with tails over its entire area, and with ermine at the front edges. A band of velvet attached to the neck under the shoulder-cape has a label 'Ede, Son & Ravenscroft

Established 1689; Robe Makers; Court Tailors; by Special Appointments to the King and Queen, 93 & 94 Chancery Lane W.C.'
Condition: velvet fragile; later white cotton lining
48.14/3 (formerly 33.219)

34 Purple velvet robe worn by Queen Mary as Princess of Wales at the Coronation of Edward VII, 1902. The train widens from the shoulders to the rounded hem, has a triple border of gold braid, and an ermine edging; it is lined with white satin and has a small ermine cape at the top, decorative pearl-trimmed cord and hooks for fastening to the dress.
The robe was worn again by Queen Mary, shortly after her own Coronation, at the Delhi Durbar of 1912, and then by Queen Elizabeth the Queen Mother at the Coronation of HM Queen Elizabeth II in 1953. During its re-wearings it has been altered at the shoulders–the original neckline, a deep V matching that of no 35, was subsequently built up into a high neckline and the fur cape was probably added at this point. The original ermine has been replaced by later imitation ermine.
Condition: good but slightly faded
57.16

35 Dress and train, worn by Queen Mary as Princess of Wales at the Coronation of Edward VII in 1902. The dress and the train are both of cream satin, lavishly embroidered; the dress has a pattern in gold and pearl festoons, and mimosa sprays, in gold and pearl appliqué and gold thread and spangles, and the train has a design of wreaths, and flowers in vases, in gold and silver strip, thread and spangles, and diamanté ornament. The dress is characteristically Edwardian in cut, with a tight-fitting, boned bodice and a full skirt curving outwards at the hem. The dressmaker's label reads 'Frederic, 14 & 15 Lower Grosvenor Place, Eaton Square, S.W.', and 'By Special Appointment to Her Majesty Queen Alexandra' and 'By Special Appointment to HRH the Princess of Wales'.
Condition: poor; soiled and fragile; cleaned and repaired in the Museum
D 207   *Plates 9a, 9b*

36 Dress worn at the Coronation of Edward VII, 1902, by Miss M. J. H. Buckland. The dress, made in the characteristic style of a fashionable Edwardian evening dress, is made of cream twilled silk, and white cotton almost covered with a leaf-pattern embroidered in gold-coloured untwisted silk worked in chain stitch; the character of this embroidery suggests an Indian origin but the lace trimming at the neck is the hand-made Buckinghamshire Point traditionally made in the East Midlands, an industry affected by machine-made lace but enjoying a brief revival. The dressmaker's label in the waist reads 'Harris & Toms, 13 Hinde Street, Manchester Square'.
Condition: rather poor; repaired in the Museum
29.165/4

37   Dress worn at the Coronation of Edward VII, 1902. This
dress, again in the style of an Edwardian evening dress, is of
cream twilled silk, white satin, white chiffon, and white lace
of various kinds – Honiton appliqué, embroidered net and
Leavers lace on the bodice, and net with applied needlepoint
lace (point de gaze) over the skirt. The dressmaker's label
reads 'Harris & Toms, 13 Hinde Street, Manchester Square'.
Condition: rather soiled and fragile; repaired in the Museum
29.165/5

38   Dress worn at the Coronation of Edward VII, 1902, by Lady
Mary Lygon. The dress is of grey satin embroidered with
sequins and diamanté ornament in a pattern of ostrich feathers.
Condition: very poor; incomplete, the lining missing, the
centre back seam unpicked
38.124

39   Wand and armband of a gold staff officer at the Coronation of
Edward VII, 1902. The wooden wand, length 30 ins, is red-
painted with gold ends; it has the royal cipher, and '1902',
'CORONATION'. The arm-band, of white cloth, is embroidered
mostly in gold thread and silver strip, with the Imperial
crown, the sword and sceptre crossed, the orb, and '1902'.
Condition: good
27.10/1, 2

The Delhi Coronation Durbar, 1903

40   The 'Peacock' dress, worn by Lady Curzon as Vicereine at
the Coronation Durbar held in Delhi in 1903. The dress is
embroidered all over with a pattern of peacock feathers in
metal thread, the eyes of the feathers of green beetles' wings.
The bodice has an elaborate jewel-like trimming of diamanté
and gilt ornament; the hem is trimmed with white roses. The
dressmaker's label reads: 'Worth PARIS'.
Condition: fair; the embroidery is tarnished but only slightly
so; the bodice has been relined and the tulle trimming at the
neck renewed
32.155   *Plate 10*

41   Panels of embroidery (2), possibly for wearing at the Delhi
Durbar. These white satin rectangles are richly embroidered
with peacocks in coiled gold and silver thread and blue and
green silk, amongst flowers in gold and silver thread and white
silk; the larger panel is shaped for a flared centre front skirt
panel, and the other panel has a stomacher and two narrow
strips the length of the skirt panel. The superb quality of this
work indicates a special occasion; its character suggests an
Indian origin, and the design and the crimped silver thread
suggest a relationship with Lady Curzon's dress (no 40). It
appears likely that the embroidery was for wear under a
peeress's robes of the traditional type (no 80).
Condition: as new
70.191

The Coronation of George V, 1911

42 Purple velvet robe worn by George V at his Coronation, 1911.
The robe is very similar to that worn by Edward VII – a cape,
ending in a long train, with a shoulder-cape and edging of
ermine and a triple border of gold braid. The front edges are
held back with ties of white satin ribbon.
Condition: fair; the gold braid is tarnished, the original ermine
has been replaced by later imitation ermine, and the satin
ribbons have been renewed
48.14/5 (formerly 33.216/1) *Plate 11*

43 Purple satin surcoat, worn by George V at his Coronation in
1911, and subsequently by George VI in 1937. The front
edges meet, and fasten with hooks and eyes; the edges have
double gold braid borders.
Condition: poor
52.71 *Plate 11*

44 Breeches worn by George V at his Coronation in 1911. The
knee-breeches are of cream satin, lined with cream twilled
silk, with gilt knee-buckles and a fly fastening at the centre
front.
Condition: fair
72.2 *Plate 11*

45 Cap of Estate, worn by King George V on his way to his
Coronation. The flat cap of crimson velvet is gathered into a
circlet of miniver, fitting the head; it is lined with white silk.
Condition: fairly good except that the centre button is missing
48.14/4 (formerly 33.219/2)

46 Girdle and stole worn by George V at his Coronation, 1911.
The stole, of gold tissue lined with crimson silk, is embroidered
with the national emblems of Great Britain and the Empire in
coloured silks with a little gold and silver thread. The girdle,
also of gold tissue lined with crimson silk, is without
embroidery.
Condition: good
52.111/1, 2 (formerly D 236) *Plate 15*

47 Coronation glove presented to George V by the Lord of the
Manor of Worksop. The glove is exactly like that presented to
Edward VII (no 25) except that the pattern of the
embroidery has become stylised into mere ornamental foliage
and the national symbols are no longer distinguishable.
Condition: good but soiled
48.14/6 (formerly 33.216/2)

48 Tracings for the embroidery on Queen Mary's Coronation
robe.
54.140/41, 45 – 80 *Plate 12*

49 Samples of embroidery for Queen Mary's Coronation robe; these include a Tudor rose, partly worked in gold thread on purple velvet, and a thistle applied to a roundel of gold tissue, and a small strip of velvet.
Condition: as new
54.140/43, 44   *Plate 14*

50 Purple velvet robe worn by Queen Mary at her Coronation, 1911. The robe is very similar to that of Queen Alexandra – a round-ended train, 18 ft by 5 ft, with shoulder-cape and edging of ermine; the original lining, to save expense, was white rabbit. The embroidered design, and its symbolism, are again not unlike the 1902 prototype; within a single border of oak leaves, roses, thistles and shamrocks a tree with the same emblems, culminating in the Queen's initial M and the Imperial Crown, represent the British Empire, the breadth and complexity of which is shown in the spreading and inter-twined roots and branches. The area above this design is scattered with roses, shamrocks and thistles. The pattern was designed by Miss Jessie Robinson, who supervised the embroidery on Queen Alexandra's robe. Like Queen Alexandra's robe, Queen Mary's was worked by HRH Princess Louise's Ladies' Work Society, for the firm of Messrs Warner of Braintree, on velvet made by Mr Cook of Sudbury; the robe was made up by Messrs Wilkinson and Sons of Maddox Street, London.
Condition: rather poor; velvet torn and fragile, embroidery tarnished, the original ermine replaced by later imitation ermine.
48.14/8 (formerly 33.217/2)   *Plates 11, 12, 13*

51 Tracings for the embroidery on Queen Mary's coronation dress.
54.140/38, 81, 82

52 Dress worn by Queen Mary for her Coronation in 1911. The dress is of cream satin, embroidered mostly in various types of gold thread, with the rose, thistle and shamrock, a border of waves at the hem representing the oceans connecting the British Empire, and the lotus and the Star of India. The lace trimming at the neck is the needlepoint type characteristic of Venetian work in the 17th century and subsequently reproduced in the 19th century in Ireland. The gold lace trimming of the sleeves is bobbin lace, also hand-made. The elaborate construction of the inside of the bodice is characteristic of the period, as is the general style of the dress, made without a waist seam. This dress is made in the style which, with a certain amount of modification of the skirt length and the material, Queen Mary was to wear for the rest of her life. In choosing this style for her Coronation dress, she has ignored the fashionable tendency towards a high-waisted style, which can be seen in the dresses worn by her six train-bearers (nos 55 and 56).

The maker's label inside the dress is that of Reville and Rossiter, the Queen's dressmakers, and they designed the dress; but the pattern was traced, and the dress fitted by Miss Jessie Robinson, who designed and supervised the embroidery for the Queen's purple velvet robe.
Condition: fragile; the dress has been relined in the Museum, and has been cleaned and restored, partly by Mrs. Karen Finch, and partly in the Museum under her supervision.
48.14/7 (formerly 33.217/1) *Plates 11, 13*

53 Designs for the embroidery of Queen Mary's coronation shoes. 54.140/2

54 Shoes worn by Queen Mary for her Coronation in 1911. The shoes are of white kid, with heels of medium height, and low fronts embroidered with a rose, thistles and shamrock in gold thread and beads. The maker's label reads 'Hook Knowles & Co. Ltd. Makers to the Royal Family, 66 & 65 New Bond Street, London'. The design was selected by Queen Mary from several drawings by Miss Jessie Robinson (no 53).
Condition: rather soiled
72.3

55 Dress worn by Lady Victoria Carrington, one of the six train-bearers to Queen Mary at her Coronation, 1911. The dress is of cream satin, with a centre front panel of beads sewn on in a trellis pattern, and a large butterfly worked in applied pearl beads over the bust, giving the impression of a high waist without any actual waist seam; there is similar butterfly decoration at the centre front hem and on the short net sleeves.
Condition: rather soiled and fragile
31.139

Plate 16

56 Dress worn by Lady Mabell Ogilvy, one of the six train-bearers to Queen Mary 1911, identical to no 55.
Condition: fair; restored in the Museum
35.164/1

57 Dress worn by Princess Mary (The Princess Royal) at the Coronation of King George V in 1911. The dress is of white chiffon over satin, with lace and satin ribbon trimming.
Condition: very fragile and soiled; washed and restored in the Museum
33.233

58 Dress worn by Lady Minto at the Coronation of George V, in 1911, and by the mother of the donor at the Delhi Durbar, in 1912. The dress, of white damask with coiled metal thread embroidery on the trained skirt, and chiffon, lace, pearl and spangle trimming on the bodice, is made in the high-waisted style fashionable by 1911. The dressmaker's label reads 'Impey, Court Dressmaker, 48 Wigmore Street'.
Condition: bodice very fragile
50.72/1

59 Uniform worn by the Page of the Master of the Horse at the Coronation of George V in 1911, and again at the Coronation of George VI in 1937; this is made in an 18th-century style and consists of a navy-blue cloth coat with lighter blue cuffs and silver braid edging and frogging at the front and cuff edges; two pairs of white stockings, black shoes, lace cravat and a sword. A label in the coat is inscribed 'Hon. F. Erskine 1911'.
Condition: good
37.152

60 Robe worn at the Coronation of George V by the Lord Mayor, Sir Thomas Vezey Strong, KCVO, KBE; a semi-circular cape of crimson velvet lined with white corded silk, gathered at the neck under an ermine shoulder-cape with three rows of tails; ermine borders at front edges, and gold cord ties with very large gold thread and yellow silk tassels. The maker's label reads 'Ede Son & Ravenscroft, Established 1689; Robe Makers, Court Tailors, by special appointments to the King & Queen. 93 & 94 Chancery Lane W.C.'; inscribed 'Alderman Sir Vezey Strong'; two white satin rosettes were received with the robe, to be used on the shoulders, to cover the attachment of the Collar of SS.
Condition; good; the lining rather soiled
A 23586

61 Wand and armband of a gold staff officer-in-waiting at the Coronation of George V, 1911. The wooden wand, length 30 ins, is red-painted with gold ends; it has the Royal cipher, and '1911', 'CORONATION'. The armband, of white cloth, is embroidered mostly in gold thread and silver strip with the Imperial Crown, the sword and sceptre crossed, the orb, and '1911'. It is almost exactly like the similar wand and armband used at the Coronation of Edward VII, 1902 (no 39).
Condition: good.
27.10/3, 4

62 Wand and armband, identical with no 61.
Condition: good; preserved in a specially-made case
57.117/6

63 Piece of material, part of that used to drape Westminster Abbey at the Coronation of George V, 1911. The fabric has a blue velvet pile on a fawn cotton background, woven with a formal foliage pattern reminiscent of 16th-century textile designs.
Condition: good
67.50

The Delhi Coronation Durbar, 1912

64   Dress worn at the Delhi Coronation Durbar, 1912. The dress
is of white satin, with a separate bodice and skirt, the bodice
trimming suggesting the fashionable high waistline, though
the skirt is fuller than those being fashionably worn in
England at the time. The front skirt panel, and the back and
sleeves of the bodice, are embroidered in green, pink and dark
red silks worked in stem and satin stitch, with a design from
the carving on the red stone palace built for Miriam Bibi, one
of the Emperor Akbar's wives. The bodice is trimmed with
bobbin lace made by Indian women, taught by the mission-
aries; it shows a mingling of the Buckinghamshire Point and
Bedfordshire Maltese styles, as well as a certain amount of
oriental influence in the design.
Condition: as new
42.26   *Plate 17*
See also no. 58

The Coronation of George VI, 1937

65   Cloth-of-gold girdle and stole worn by King George VI at
his Coronation, 1937. Both are lined with crimson satin;
the stole is embroidered with the national emblems in coloured
silks and has fringed ends; the girdle is embroidered with gold
thread in an arabesque pattern similar to that on the supertunica of Edward VII.
Condition: good
54.77/1, 2

66   Coronation glove, presented to George VI by the Lord of the
Manor of Worksop; identical to that presented to Edward VII
in 1902 (no 25), but lacking the glove-case.
Condition: good
54.77/3

67   Purple velvet robe worn by Queen Elizabeth the Queen
Mother, at the Coronation of George VI, 1937. The robe is
similar to those of Queen Alexandra and Queen Mary, with an
ermine shoulder-cape and borders and a rounded end, but
it is lined with white satin instead of fur. There are decorative
gold cords for fastening the robe to the shoulders. The tip
and the borders are embroidered in gold thread with national
emblems – oak leaves, rose, thistle, shamrock, leek, lotus,
maple leaves, fern leaves and mimosa. There is also the
Imperial Crown and two interlaced 'E's'. The maker's label
reads 'EDE & RAVENSCROFT Founded 1689 Robe Makers Court
Tailors By Appointment to the King, the Queen, the Prince
of Wales 93 & 94 Chancery Lane W.C.2'.
Condition: good
52.17/1   *Plate 20*

68 Dress worn by Queen Elizabeth the Queen Mother at the Coronation of George VI, 1937. The dress is of white satin embroidered with gold thread, diamanté and spangles with roses, thistles, shamrocks, leeks, lotus, maple leaves, fern leaves and mimosa. It shows the cross-cutting characteristic of 1930s dressmaking, and has short satin sleeves and long hanging sleeves of net with applied needlepoint (point de gaze).
Condition: good, some lace missing from one of the sleeves
52.17/2   *Plate 19*

69 Shoes worn by Queen Elizabeth the Queen Mother at the Coronation of George VI, 1937. The shoes are of white satin with high heels and low fronts, embroidered with oak leaves and thistles in gold thread. The maker's label reads 'Jack Jacobus Ltd. 39/45 Shaftesbury Avenue, London W.'.
Condition: good
52.17/3

70 Purple velvet robe worn by Princess Elizabeth (later Queen Elizabeth II) at the Coronation of her father, King George VI, in 1937. The robe is a miniature version of that worn by Queen Mary as Princess of Wales in 1902 (no 34) and subsequently worn by her again as Queen at the Delhi Durbar of 1912, and yet again as Queen Dowager in 1937; this was, incidentally, the first coronation at which a Queen Dowager was present. The presence of the two young Princesses (Princess Elizabeth was 10, Princess Margaret 6) in the Abbey procession was another innovation. The maker's label (Ede & Ravenscroft) is exactly like that on the robe worn by Queen Elizabeth the Queen Mother (no 67) but is inscribed 'Her Royal Highness Princess Elizabeth'.
Condition: good
52.18/1

71 Dress worn by Princess Elizabeth at the Coronation of her father, King George VI, in 1937. The long dress is made of white cotton machine lace (Leavers) with a gold waistband and gold bows down the centre front, and a satin under-dress with the maker's label 'Smith & Co., 193 Sloane Street, S.W.'
Condition: good, but the lace is very limp, the dress apparently having been laundered
52.18/3

72 Coronet, gilt metal, worn by Princess Elizabeth at the Coronation of her father, King George VI, in 1937.
Condition: good
52.18/2

73 Purple velvet robe worn by Princess Margaret at the Coronation of her father, King George VI, in 1937. Similar to, but smaller than, that worn by Princess Elizabeth (no 70).
Condition: good
52.19/1

74   Dress worn by Princess Margaret at the Coronation of her father, King George VI, in 1937. Similar to, but smaller than, that worn by Princess Elizabeth on the same occasion (no 71). Condition: good but the lace is limp, apparently as a result of laundering

52.19/3   *Plate 18*

75   Coronet, gilt metal, worn by Princess Margaret at the Coronation of her father, King George VI, in 1937. Similar to that worn by Princess Elizabeth on the same occasion (no 72). Condition: good

52.19/2

76   Coronet, silver-gilt, with alternating strawberry leaves and fleurs-de-lis, crimson velvet crown-cap and cream silk lining. It was made for the Marquess of Carisbrooke, grandson of Queen Victoria, in 1937, and was worn for the Coronation of George VI and of HM Queen Elizabeth II in 1953. The form differs from that usually worn by the rank as it incorporates the fleurs-de-lis found on the coronets of royalty. Condition: good

60.66/1

77   Dress worn by Princess Marina of Kent (then the Duchess of Kent) at the Coronation of King George VI, in 1937. The dress is of fawn lamé woven with a pattern of feathers which is emphasised by lavish embroidery with spangles, beads and rhinestones. The low-necked, short-sleeved dress is cut with a slight train, in the clinging style of the 1930s but without the usual bias cutting; the heavy embroidery required the support of material cut on the straight, and its weight ensures the close fit so essential to the 1930s line. The dressmaker's label reads 'Modele Molyneux, Grosvenor St., Made in England'. Condition: good

68.146/1   *Plate 21*

78   Blue velvet robe worn by Princess Helena Victoria at the Coronation of King George VI, 1937, and subsequently by Princess Marie Louise at the Coronation of HM Queen Elizabeth II, 1953. The train widens slightly from a pleated top, with hooks for fastening to the dress, to a rounded end; it is lined with and trimmed with appliqué decoration of silver lamé.

Condition: fairly good, but crushed and slightly faded in parts

57.38/1

79   Cloak for one of the royal chaplains at the Coronation of King George VI, in 1937; a full-length collarless cloak of scarlet cloth, lined with white silk, the neck fastening with red and white silk cords. The maker's label 'Ede and Ravenscroft' is the same as those on the robes of Queen Elizabeth the Queen Mother and the Princesses; it is inscribed 'Rev. A. R. Fuller'. Condition: as new

68.97

80   Coronation robes of a peeress (kirtle, train and cape) and
coronet, worn by the Dowager Countess of Airlie at the
Coronation of King George V, in 1911, and again, with some
alteration, at the Coronation of King George VI, in 1937. The
robes include a train of crimson velvet, with an ermine
shoulder-cape, with three rows of ermine tails to indicate the
rank of countess, an ermine border with a narrow gold braid
inner border, a white silk lining, and gold cords for attaching
the robe to the shoulders; there is also a fitted crimson velvet
kirtle, the short sleeves with two rows of white fur and fur-
edged vandyked points at the edge. The kirtle is open down
the front, meeting at the waist, and has a white satin
stomacher and separate skirt-panel, both with gold
embroidery.
The coronet is the type worn by a countess; eight silver balls
raised on points alternating with eight silver-gilt strawberry
leaves on a circlet, with a miniver rim and a silk-lined crimson
velvet crown cap with a gold lace finial. Made by R. & S.
Garrard, 1910/11.
Condition: good, but so altered (presumably for the 1937
wearing) that the robes must be regarded as belonging to the
1937 occasion rather than that of 1911.
37.135

The Coronation of H.M. Queen Elizabeth II, 1953

81   Purple velvet cap from the interior of St. Edward's Crown,
worn by HM Queen Elizabeth II at her Coronation, 1953. The
cap consists of a circle of purple velvet, pleated round the edge
to form a flat cap-shape.
Condition: fair; lining missing
59.7/1

82   Purple velvet cap from the interior of the Imperial State
Crown, worn by HM Queen Elizabeth II at her Coronation,
1953. The cap is like the last, but smaller, and complete with
a white silk lining, and press-studs just above the inside edge.
Condition: good
59.7/2

83   Dress worn by HRH Princess Margaret, Countess of Snowdon
at the Coronation of HM Queen Elizabeth II in 1953. The
dress is of heavy white satin, embroidered in a flower and
festoon pattern with pearls, rhinestones, spangles and silver
thread; the neckline is wide and square and there are no
sleeves. The very full skirt with its elaborate stiffening and
support inside, and the built-in bust support, are characteristic
of 1950s haute couture; the maker's label reads 'Hartnell
London Paris'.
Condition: good
68.6/1   *Plate 22*

84 Kilt jacket, worn by HRH Prince Michael of Kent, as a boy, at the Coronation of HM Queen Elizabeth II, 1953. The jacket is made in the traditional Highland style, of dark green woollen cloth (barathea).
Condition: good
69.113/1

85 Dress worn by Princess Marie Louise at the Coronation of HM Queen Elizabeth II, 1953. The dress is of pale grey satin woven with a silver pattern; it has a V-neck back and front, and a draped cross-over bodice, cut in one with short sleeves, and pleated into the shoulders and draped waistband. The full skirt has pleats at the back, sewn down to hip level. The style of the dress, made for an older wearer than the Hartnell dress of Princess Margaret (no 83) is reminiscent of the later 1940s rather than the 1950s.
Condition: good
57.38/4

86 Dress worn at the Coronation of HM Queen Elizabeth II, 1953, by Lady Hutton, CBE. The dress is of white and gold material woven with a small pattern of tulips; the tight-fitting bodice with boned lining, the sleeveless style with shawl collar, and the full skirt pleated to the waist are entirely characteristic of fashionable evening wear at this period.
Condition: good
60.13   *Plate 25*

87 Coronation robes (kirtle, train and coronet) worn at the Coronation of George VI, 1937 by Gertrude, Countess of Dudley (formerly Gertie Millar) and at the Coronation of HM Queen Elizabeth II, 1953, by Countess Jowitt, together with the dress (no 88). The train is very similar to that of the Dowager Countess of Airlie (no 80), worn 1911 and again 1937, but without the inner gold border. The kirtle too is similar but the sleeves have a third broader edging of fur instead of the vandyked edge, and the front has no attached stomacher or separate front skirt panel, as in 1953 it was worn over the dress (no 88). The many hooks inside the front edges above the waist suggest that in 1937 it was worn similarly to no 80. The maker's label reads 'Contessa Ltd., 116 Knightsbridge S.W.1'.
The coronet is similar to but larger than no 80. Hall mark 1936/37. In red leather box lined with white satin.
Condition: good
64.64/1   *Plate 23*

88 Dress worn by Countess Jowitt at the Coronation of HM
Queen Elizabeth II, 1953. The dress is of gold and white
fabric, woven with a fairly small leaf pattern. The style is
slim-fitting, with a straight top edge and supporting shoulder-
straps. The maker's label reads 'Victor Stiebel, at Jacqmar,
16 Grosvenor St., London W.1'. A white silk bag with gold
and silver lace decoration, and long white kid gloves, and a
tiara of gold beads, were also used, and are preserved with the
dress.
Condition: good
64.64/2

89 Coronation robe and cap of estate worn by Enid, Lady
Burnham, CBE, JP, at the Coronation of HM Queen Elizabeth
II, 1953. The robes (nos 80 and 87) are of the traditional type;
this is in a new style designed by Norman Hartnell in
conjunction with the Earl Marshall, for peeresses with newer
titles who did not possess robes worn by their ancestors. The
robe consists of one garment only (instead of the traditional
kirtle and train); it has a fur cape-collar and no sleeves, and it
fits to and is open below the waist. Like the traditional type it
is of crimson velvet, bordered with white fur and lined with
white silk. The cape has two rows of ermine tails, indicating
the rank of baroness. The stiff round cap of estate, of velvet
edged with fur and trimmed with gold braid, is an alternative
to the coronet.
Condition: good
L 25   *Plate 24*

90 Dress worn by Enid, Lady Burnham at the Coronation of
HM Queen Elizabeth II, 1953; the dress is of white satin
woven with small lions and unicorns outlined in gold. The
fitted boned bodice is trimmed with complex drapes typical of
evening wear in the late 1940s and early 1950s and the broad
pleated shoulder straps form a low square neckline. The
fullness in the skirt is concentrated at the back which is cut
from a semi-circle, and the hips are accentuated by the addition
of shallow floating panels below the back waist. The maker's
label reads 'MARSHALL & SNELGROVE LONDON'. Worn under
crimson velvet robe (no 89).
Condition: good
72.30

Coronation Costume and Accessories 1685-1953

CORRECTIONS

The following entries should be added to the catalogue under the coronations indicated.

91   The Coronation of Edward VII, 1902

Shoes worn by Queen Mary as Princess of Wales at the Coronation of Edward VII, 1902. The shoes are of white kid, with low fronts and imitation bows embroidered with clear glass and gilt beads; the heels are of medium height.
Condition: good but soiled and lining fragile
D.204–5
Given by Queen Mary

92   Coronation robes of a peeress (dress and train) worn by Anne, Countess of Moray at the Coronation of Edward VII, 1902. The robes include a train of crimson velvet with narrow ermine edging and an ermine shoulder-cape with three rows of tails denoting rank; gold cords with tassels are attached at the shoulders. The dress (separate bodice and skirt) is of crimson velvet with ermine edgings, except for the centre front (bodice and skirt) sections which are of white corded silk embroidered with gold and silver thread, pearls, spangles, diamanté and lace; the dressmaker's label reads 'Jessica Rice, 49 Ebury Street'.
Condition: good apart from very fragile linings; alterations at the back of the dress suggest a later wearing, possibly in 1911
73.81
Purchased at Christie, Manson and Woods

93   The Coronation of George V, 1911

Gloves worn by Queen Mary at her Coronation in 1911. Long white kid gloves with the wrist-opening fastened with buttons and buttonholes; the crown and royal cypher are embroidered above the wrist in gold and silver thread.
Condition: soiled and stained, the metal thread tarnished
48.14/9 (formerly 33.217/3, D.393)
Given by Queen Mary

The Coronation of George VI, 1937

94 Dress worn by Princess Marie Louise at the Coronation of King George VI, 1937. The dress is of pale grey satin woven with chrysanthemums and foliage in pale pink and green; the flowers down the centre front are embellished with embroidery of beads, sequins and diamanté. The bodice is softly draped at the front with a V-neck and deep cape sleeves; the semi-circular skirt falls into a short train at the back. The maker's label reads 'Woollands, Knightsbridge'.
Condition: good
57.38/3
Given by HRH The Duchess of Gloucester

95 Dress worn by Princess Helena Victoria at the Coronation of King George VI, 1937. The dress is of heavy silver machine lace over a silver lamé underdress lined with pink silk; it has a V-neck at front and back, the armholes are trimmed with fine silver lace, and the skirt extends into a train at the back. The style of the dress, straight and without a waist seam, is essentially still that of the previous decade. The maker's label reads 'Reville, London'. Worn with blue velvet train (no 78).
Condition: good
57.38/2
Given by HRH The Duchess of Gloucester

96 Coronation robes of a peeress (kirtle, train and cape) worn by the Marchioness of Carisbrooke at the Coronation of King George VI, 1937, and at the Coronation of HM Queen Elizabeth II, 1953. The robes are of crimson velvet trimmed with imitation ermine and are virtually identical to those worn by the Countess of Dudley and Countess Jowitt (no 87). The cape, however, has three and a half rows of tails to denote the higher rank. The maker's label in the kirtle reads 'Modèle Sidon, 24 Sloane Street, S.W.1; that in the train reads 'Ede and Ravenscroft Ltd. Founded 1689 Robe Makers Court Tailors by Appointment to the King, the Queen and Queen Mary 93 and 94 Chancery Lane W.C.2' and is inscribed 'Marchioness of Carisbrooke'.
Condition: good
60.66/2
Given by Queen Victoria Eugenie of Spain

Catalogue entry 60 should be amended as follows:

60 The robe held by the Museum is presumably that worn by the Lord Mayor at post-Coronation ceremonies when entertaining the King and Queen in the City. For the actual coronation ceremony he wore a robe of crimson velvet with four horizontal bands of gold braid and miniver.

LONDON: HER MAJESTYS STATIONERY OFFICE : 1973

Acknowledgements

Acknowledgements and thanks are due to the following for help in the compilation of this catalogue: Mr Geoffrey de Bellaigue, Colonel Sir Thomas Butler, Lady Paula Chapman, the Worshipful Company of Glovers, Mr John Morley, Mr Derek Rogers and the National Museum of Wales. Thanks are also due to the London Museum staff who contributed to this catalogue, in particular Miss Kay Staniland, who succeeded Miss Zillah Halls as Curator of Costume, and Miss Davina Fennemore.

List of Sources

Gifts

HM The Queen 12 (crown-frame) 67 68 69 70 71 72 81 82
HM Queen Alexandra 29 30 31 32
HRH The Duchess of Gloucester 78 85
TRH The Duke of Kent, Princess Alexandra of Kent, Prince
  Michael of Kent 77
HRH Prince Michael of Kent 84
HRH Princess Margaret, The Countess of Snowdon 73 74 75
  83
HM Queen Mary 13 14 19 23 24 25 26 33 39 42 43 45 46 47 50
  52 61
HM Queen Victoria Eugenie of Spain 76
The Dowager Countess of Airlie CBE 56 80
Lady Benson 64
Miss M. J. H. Buckland 36 37
Enid Lady Burnham CBE JP 90
Lady Cory 17 18
Sir H Creedy GCB KCVO 62
The Rt Hon the Earl of Cromer KCIE GCVO 16
Lady Victoria Forrester 55
The Rt Hon the Earl of Granard KP 59
Lt Gen Sir Thomas Hutton KCIE 86
The Countess Jowitt 87 88
The Rev A Lea-Wilson 8
Lady Maufe 79
Dr J A Pratt-Johnson 11
Mrs Graham Rees-Mogg 12 (circlet and cap)
Miss J. Robinson 22 27 28 48 49 51 53
Mrs A G C Sheppard 7
Col R H G O Spence CBE 58
Lady Vezey Strong 60
Lt Col the Hon Henry Trefusis 38
Mrs M Turner 6

Loans

HM The Queen 3 21 35 57 65 66
HM Queen Elizabeth the Queen Mother 34
Lord Amherst of Hackney 2 4 10
The Rt Hon the Earl of Ancaster TD 5
The Rt Hon The Lord Cullen of Ashbourne 20
Enid Lady Burnham 89
Lady Ravensdale 40

Purchases

E T Biggs & Sons Ltd 1
Miss H M Lancaster 63
Messrs Sotheby 15

Anonymous Sources

9 41 44 54

Bibliography

Sandford, J. 1687. *History of the Coronation of James II.* Thomas Newcomb.

Younghusband, Sir G. and **Davenport, C.** 1919. *The Crown Jewels of England.* Cassell & Co.

Holmes, M. R. 1936. The Crowns of England. *Archaeologia* vol. LXXXVI.

Perkins, Dr. J. 1937. *The Crowning of the Sovereign.* Methuen.

The Times. 1937. *Crown and Empire.*

Illustrated London News. May 1937. Coronation Edition.

Broad, L. 1952. *Crowns, Queens and Coronations.* Hutchinson.

Churchill, R. S. 1953. *The Story of the Coronation.* Verschoyle.

Tanner, L. 1952. *The History of the Coronation.* Pitkin.

The Daily Express. 1953. *Coronation Glory.*

Sitwell, Major Gen. H. D. W. 1953. *The Crown Jewels.* Dropmore Press Ltd.

Illustrated London News. June 1953. Coronation Edition.

Country Life. June 1953. Coronation Edition.

The Queen. June 1953. Coronation Edition.

Holmes, M. R. The Vanished Crown of Mary of Modena. *Illustrated London News.* 30 June, 1956.

Printed in England for Her Majesty's Stationery Office by Headley Brothers Ltd., 109 Kingsway, London WC2B 6PX and Ashford Kent   Dd 503879 K60